T0208800

A GUIDE FOR NURSE CASE MANAGERS

A GUIDE FOR NURSE CASE MANAGERS

CHARLOTTE COX

IUNIVERSE, INC.
NEW YORK   BLOOMINGTON

A Guide for Nurse Case Managers

*The information, ideas, and suggestions in this book are not intended
as a substitute for professional medical advice. Before following any
suggestions contained in this book, you should consult your personal
physician. Neither the author nor the publisher shall be liable or
responsible for any loss or damage allegedly arising as a consequence of
your use or application of any information or suggestions in this book.*

iUniverse books may be ordered through booksellers or by contacting:

*iUniverse
1663 Liberty Drive
Bloomington, IN 47403
www.iuniverse.com
1-800-Authors (1-800-288-4677)*

*Because of the dynamic nature of the Internet, any Web addresses or links
contained in this book may have changed since publication and may no longer be
valid. The views expressed in this work are solely those of the author and do not
necessarily reflect the views of the publisher, and the publisher hereby disclaims
any responsibility for them.*

*ISBN: 978-1-4502-3855-7 (sc)
ISBN: 978-1-4502-3856-4 (ebk)*

Printed in the United States of America

iUniverse rev. date: 9/17/2010

CONTENTS

DISCLAIMER

This book is written for use only as a guide to those new to, or who may be interested in, the practice field of nursing case management. Seasoned nurse case managers will also benefit from the guidelines, tools, and tips for helping with clients presented herein.

This book should be used only as an insightful guide to your practice and should not be taken as an ultimate resource. You are urged to read and to learn from the information presented. Please take advantage of other resources on this subject and follow the links provided for further research.

Case management is a field evolving, and nurses learn daily from helping those who need our services. The author presents ideas relative to the case management field at the time of print. Discussions of guidelines, tips, and tools presented are those of the author, as related to experiences encountered, research, and ideas formulated over time. Note: efforts were aimed at making this book as complete and accurate as possible. Therefore, note again that this book is to be used as a general guide.

The author shall not be held liable or have responsibility to any individual person or entity for any loss alleged or damages caused, directly or indirectly, by the information presented. All persons referred to in the book are fictional.

Preface—Note to the Reader

Many of us entered into a chosen nursing specialty once out of school. We hoped to do our very best within our careers. You mastered the education and the clinical internships, and then you entered the workforce. Take a moment and reflect on that first job you landed.

Remember the anxieties you experienced? *Will I know everything in order to do well? Do I really have the skills for this job? How will I ever remember all of this information?*

I've worked in health care for over thirty years. My career has spanned many areas, including providing care to nursing home residents, delivering medical and surgical care, providing nursing services in intensive care units, delivering care to respiratory-compromised clients, extensive nursing in cardiac units, managing a cardiac step-down unit, and in the past decade, perfecting my skills within the case management field. I've enjoyed all aspects of the nursing fields chosen. But I especially enjoy nursing case management and the position of a nurse case manager.

The knowledge I have obtained with the continued education I have received since graduating helps to motivate me to perform at my best in whatever field I pursue. I continually strive to attain my greatest potential in servicing others entrusted to my care.

As you reflect on your first job, let me tell you a little more about those earlier years. At fifteen years old, I began work. I worked weekends in a small city nursing home. My mother was the chief cook, and with her connections, I was hired. Don't ever underestimate the influence that family or friends have in your attempts to be hired.

I don't recall having a lot of responsibility except to wash, dry, and fold about twenty loads of laundry while working the night shift. After the eight hours of orientation, I was left alone to fulfill the job duties assigned.

Of course, the duties were basic and easy to comprehend. You may have had a similar first job. No worries, no sweat. You mature and complete the required education of your desired occupation; you then reenter the workforce.

Circumstances are different for many of us. What is the difference, you ask? Maybe you have a desire to be all you can and do it better than anyone else. Ah, competition in the field? Not really. Do you hunger for the perfect job? Is your heart with infant care, emergency medical services, or intensive care nursing? Do you prefer clinic nursing, home health care, hospice, or taking the time to get to know your elderly patients?

You begin to set goals in order to achieve success in your field. And yet, you want what most of us want ... to simply do a great job no matter the circumstances.

Have I got your attention? Now you might be asking, "What has this got to do with being a nurse case manager?" Well, remember the anxieties you felt as a student of nursing? That first day of clinical should stir memories. Some good memories, hopefully, will begin to fill your mind too. See one, do one, teach one! Remember?

Early in my career, I was assigned to give a bed bath to a young man who had been involved in a car wreck. His arms were broken and casted, and one leg was wrapped in dressings marking an injury sustained. He was indeed young, and yet so was I. Here I was nursing in my late teens and to top it all off, providing care to one whose age matched closely to mine. *Wow!* Sweating and avoiding eye contact, I completed the task and left the room with my face beet red. I had survived!

Another situation commanded insight into dispensing medication. Nervous about what my instructor might ask, I prepared in advance the answers to potential queries. What are the drug's adverse effects? Name the indications for giving this drug to your patient. Can you recite the usual dosage? Nursing implications? Are there any contraindications to the dispensing of this drug? Can you see where this is leading?

Before the instructor's last question, I was on a roll with information about my client's medication that would stop a professor dead in his or her tracks. Afterward, my confidence level peeked as I if I had climbed Mount Everest. You know the feeling of mastering a technique, the adrenaline rush, and, ah, the satisfaction gained.

As you embark upon the field of nursing case management, you undoubtedly will have a whole new set of anxieties. *How will I learn all this insurance information?* You take notice when you overhear co-workers discussing dismissal plans, state and federal regulations, and you ask, *What the heck is everyone talking about?*

How will I ever remember all of this information?

The orientation is nothing like what you've encountered at the bedside—insurance, clinical reviews, dismissal planning, length-of-stay issues, Medicare, and so much information day to day. Your head is spinning, and you may wonder, *What have I gotten myself into as a nurse case manager?*

Within the following pages, you will gain easy insight into this field called case management. The information will help to prepare you for the role of nurse case manager. Whether you practice in a hospital setting, a clinic, or at a health plan office, this book, *A Guide for Nurse Case Managers*, will be a handy reference for the days and months ahead.

Whether you are a new case manager, a student, or a seasoned nurse needing a refresher about job basics, this book will help to guide your practice, provide valuable tips and reference tools, and help you with proven organizational ideas. You will find many books and CDs available on the market that discuss nursing case management. Many books outline in great detail the concepts of case management and insurance practices and compile an in-depth look at the field. This book is a condensed, user-friendly reference tool for new nurses entering the field of nursing case management.

As the chapters unfold, the nurse case manager role is defined. We will discuss how the nurse case manager utilizes the nursing process with patient assessment and medication assistance. You will also find valuable information pertaining to insurance precertification and authorization. Information basics pertaining to Medicare and Medicaid with an emphasis on utilization practices are lightly covered.

Yes, you *will* need a library of information at your fingertips to further your knowledge regarding the practice of case management. This book is *the* key reference to jump-start your practice and to build understanding of the concepts you will need for a successful career. My hope is that you come away with vital information necessary for you to step right into the nursing case manager role your first day on the job.

Therefore, let's begin the journey toward building a successful career as a nurse case manager within the field of case management.

Acknowledgments

It seems only a few years ago that I dove into the field of case management. Actually, ten years have passed, and I'm still learning every day. The avenue of nursing is never boring, as challenges occur daily. Patients and their families need guidance with so many aspects of care that a nurse case manager's work is never done.

As a nurse in this field, a case manager brings a set of skills that easily bridges into another specialty of nursing. Effective communication between health team members, exceptional problem-solving skills, and the clinical knowledge acquired through years of nursing practice help the new case manager become an active leader within this interesting field of nursing. I have worked alongside many former nurse managers who now work as nurse case managers.

Many of my colleagues have contributed their knowledge and valuable information to the ideas presented in this manual. Without our peers, we may not take the less easy but more rewarding path. I've been challenged and have a passion to improve policies, practice guidelines, and overall communication to unlock the barriers encountered on a daily basis. Barriers encountered within the entire health system including process failures involving the healthcare team, and also social issues involving the patient and family.

Charlotte Cox

Special thanks to Robin Wood, a nurse colleague, for her friendship during the writing of this book. Her words of wisdom and encouragement have made a huge impact on the success of my career in case management. Also sincere thanks to the publishing staff at iUniverse.

Heartfelt thanks to everyone who made this all possible and to my family for allowing me the time necessary to complete this project.

CHAPTER 1

THE CASE MANAGER ROLE

DEFINITION OF CASE MANAGEMENT

Let's begin by defining *case management*. The Commission for Case Manager Certification (CCM) states, "Case Management is a collaborative process that assesses, plans, implements, coordinates, monitors, and evaluates the options and services required to meet an individual's health needs, using communication and available resources to promote quality, cost-effective outcomes."[1]

You're hired as nurse case manager. As you begin this new career in nursing, questions surface about the role. Beginning with the very first day of orientation, terms, such as *utilization*, *discharge planning*, and *insurance contracts*, heighten your interest. This verbiage is only the start of a new language of nursing. You also hear discussions regarding length-of-stay issues, variance tracking reports, and insurance authorizations, as the list continues.

---

1. Case Management Society of America, "What Is a Case Manager?" http:/www.ccmcertification.org/ (accessed November 18, 2009).

1

It isn't long before you figure out that case management is unlike any other nursing field you've experienced. Wow! This is such a new avenue of nursing for you and many others.

Nurse Case Manager Functions

The nurse case manager is the one person who guides the patient through the health system. Service areas include hospital case management, worker's compensation, health plans, disease management, outpatient care, military programs, and agencies providing services to the homebound patient.[2] Many avenues exist, allowing the case manager to assess and plan for life-care changes for any age group.

Depending on the facility program, social workers and case managers may perform similar duties in providing case management. The nurse case managers educate the patient with vital information regarding their disease process and expected outcomes, while coordinating services as identified in patient/family interviewing.

Brief Overview of the Case Manager Utilization of the Nursing Process

A thorough assessment reveals actual or potential patient needs for which the nurse case manager can then begin planning and coordinating services as applicable. Handy assessment tools used during the interviewing process will help the case manager organize caseloads. Once all parties agree on the needs identified and the plan outlined to meet the needs, the case manager will then coordinate and implement the individualized case plan.

This nursing process requires excellent communication across the continuum of care among health-care providers. Don't forget to include the immediate family members and significant others,

---

2.　C. M. Mullahy and D. K. Jensen, *Student Guide to Accompany The Case Manager's Handbook*, 3rd ed. (Sudbury, MA: Jones and Bartlett, 2004).

who play an important role in helping our patients meet their care needs. As a patient advocate, the nurse case manager seeks quality, cost-effective resources in order to meet the identified care needs.

Just remember to follow the Health Insurance Portability and Accountability Act (HIPAA) guidelines during initial interviews in discussing care needs and discharge/home care plans. This act, which was passed in 1996, allows the federal government to regulate certain aspects of the health insurance industry. It also addresses the rights of employees, patient privacy/confidentiality standards, coding/transactions, and oversight of insured and noninsured clients.[3]

Once the case plan is implemented, the nurse case manager follows up to ensure the patient care needs are indeed met. This process includes coordinating insurance updates and selected agency/facility input. An evaluation process is vital to ensure the intended outcome is successful.

If the plan fails or is inadequate to fully meet the identified patient needs, the nurse case manager starts over. The process begins with reassessment followed by planning, implementation, and evaluation. Don't fret; many patient care plans change in midstream or as needs change in cases involving long-term medical disease processes. View this curvature as a challenge to sharpen your skills within the field of case management.

Patients and families are grateful that the nurse case manager is coordinating the hospital discharge plan or home plan. She or he is connecting them with community resources necessary to ensure care needs are met in a timely manner. Using proven methods to secure the best possible services for your clients enhances your credibility within the profession. Strive toward providing exceptional service and gaining client trust, and others will want to follow in your steps.

---

3.   P. R. Kongstvedt, *Managed Care, What It Is and How It Works*, 2nd ed. (Sudbury, MA: Jones and Bartlett, 2004).

Charlotte Cox

Tip—*Just remember to follow the Health Insurance Portability and Accountability Act guidelines during initial interviews and when discussing care needs and discharge/home care plans.*

Let's begin to delve into the tools necessary for your success within the field of case management. The following is only meant to help guide your practice and should be community tailored to address the clients served. What may seem ideal for one part of the country, in reality, may not be suited for your neck of the woods.

Individual care planning involves researching the community resources available. Take a few moments to consider the various types (homeless, low-income, military, insured, etc.) of clients served. A wise nurse case manager does the preparatory work necessary to best serve those patients and families needing guidance and care planning.

CHAPTER 2

CARE PLANNING PROCESSES

CARE PLANNING GUIDELINES

Most health-care facilities utilize practice guidelines in providing quality care to their clients served. These practice guidelines help to guide the health team with the management and delivery of care.

The primary focus is always the patient. As with facility processes implemented, care planning processes are a focus in nurse case management. Hospital departments have unique guidelines and policies outlined in order for employees to understand the expectations within their work environment. Likewise, utilization and case management departments follow a plan that all case managers and secretarial staff must understand in order to comply.

Any process should be looked at from various angles to determine the most appropriate path to achievement of the desired outcomes. Examining outcomes helps us measure the delivery and quality of care provided, thus promoting patient safety as a number-one priority. Sound familiar?

Tip—*Specific short-term and long-term goals are outlined by the nurse case manager in order to help the patient achieve these goals before dismissal from a hospital setting.*

In addition, familiar terms, such as *nursing care plans* or *clinical pathways*, may pop into your head. Nursing of the past, present, and future will always be guided in any clinical practice area. Some form of a care plan will guide the health-care team in providing holistic care to the patients. No matter the field of nursing practiced, there is a standard of care to uphold, a professional standard of conduct expected, and a desire to continue the Florence Nightingale basic traditional art and science of nursing in all of us.[4]

Care plans focus on the documentation of care provided in a narrative form. The nurse case manager outlines specific short-term and long-term goals to help the patient achieve these goals before being dismissed to go home from a hospital setting. Short-term goals may include specifics as to stabilization of a medical crisis, a normalization of lab values, or a focus in resolving the acute illness.

We see the long-term goals while helping patients to a achieve a maximal level in quality of life, returning a chronic disease process to baseline, focusing on preventative measures, and empowering clients to become managers of their own health. Did I say to empower the client? Yes, indeed!

Patients and families in today's world of communicative avenues thrive on obtaining the knowledge and the best of every available health-care technology to overcome acute, chronic, and debilitating diseases. Armed with information and literature from the Internet, the media, and social contacts, clients end up becoming their own advocates in promoting their agendas for maintaining quality health care. As we in health care are

4.   Florence Nightingale, *Notes on Nursing* (New York, NY: Barnes & Noble Books, 2003).

increasingly aware, the "I want" or "I need" may not necessarily be the appropriate standard of care for the illness or disease diagnosed.

It takes a wise and knowledgeable medical provider to discern the best practice and path to pursue with the client's treatment plan. At times, honesty is the best policy. Unfortunately, some clients don't want to hear a proposed plan that doesn't meet with their satisfaction or agenda.

Tip—*Just remember to follow these basic steps (our nursing process), which include assessing, identifying needs, determining objectives/goals, developing an action plan, implementing/coordinating the plan, and evaluating the plan.*

In some cases, the clients will pursue another provider for a second opinion, a third opinion, and so on until they achieve their own goals. Don't take it personally, because it is not. Patients have the right to follow what they feel they must do in order to see the other options available. Unfortunately, some pursue what they want regardless of what is recommended or the costs involved.

The following practice guidelines are exactly what any nurse case manager needs in order to function effectively when working with patients and families. How do you get involved? Many avenues exist for case management services.

Your referrals may come from a physician's office, a home health nurse, an insurance carrier, hospital staff, the emergency center, or urgent care, or the patient and family members may enlist your services. Depending on your practice setting and the referral process in your agency or facility, the nurse case manager is available to assist and coordinate any services related to patient care.

Just remember to follow these basic steps (our nursing process):

- Assess
- Identify needs

- Determine objectives/goals
- Develop an action plan
- Implement/coordinate plan
- Evaluate plan

Before you know it, the nursing case management process becomes second nature in your daily interactions. The practice guidelines are broken into basic steps for easy reference (refer to Quick Reference Tool #3, Case Management Patient Needs Assessment Guide).

PATIENT NEEDS ASSESSMENT GUIDE

We begin with reviewing the process of the patient needs assessment guide. As mentioned earlier, a thorough patient assessment is crucial to the identification of any real or actual care needs. The *initial patient assessment* is the in-depth data collection process to identify those needs in order to develop a comprehensive nursing case management plan (refer to Quick Reference Tool #4, Patient Needs Assessment Tool).

Assessed items should include the patient's demographics, phone contact information, employer contact information, insurance plan, medical diagnosis and pertinent medical history, specific self-care/assistance requirements, any current agency support/services, and stated perceived patient/family concerns. Remember to block at least thirty to sixty minutes to complete this initial information-gathering process. The assessment tool can be easily filed for future reference.

Once the initial assessment is completed, the case manager moves on to the next step, which is to *identify any real or potential needs*. You've gathered important information with your patient over the past hour and have likely put your contact at ease. Now is the time to focus on what exactly the perceived problem or need is. After all, you need to clarify why you're involved with the case. Allow the patient to verbalize any concerns.

You may hear problems voiced, such as a need for caregiver assistance in the home, equipment needs, insurance questions regarding coverage of services, inability to maintain therapy due to the costs of medications, guardianship issues, family conflict, and social issues. These social issues may involve living conditions, homeless concerns, paying for rent/utilities, etc.

Be prepared to direct the conversation to specific concerns, as some may trail off on unrelated issues. Specific concerns voiced help to further identify the need for case management services. Or, if not preempted, you may find yourself in the middle of a family squabble that you can't do anything to resolve. Just remember to politely listen and be supportive. List the concern objectively on your assessment form.

The second step is to correctly *identify the patient need* as perceived by the patient. Review the compiled data, and note the perceived concern identified above. Case management services will focus on the identified patient need you list. At this time, you may notice the perceived concern or need is different or could possibly be the same as the one you identified.

For instance, patient Joe Johns may seem to need home health care or home equipment based on the information provided. Yet, after conferring with Joe, you also identify he lives alone and is unable to meet his self-care needs even with enlisted agency assistance. Hence, Joe needs twenty-four-hour care, and a home plan may not be a realistic option at this time.

Once you and your client agree on the problem or a need that requires your services, outline the *objectives and goals* for the process. The case manager will strive toward accomplishment of these goals. Include short-term or long-term goals to assist your clients to successful case management. State the goals, and have the patient also restate his or her understanding of the objectives that you will strive to achieve on his or her behalf.

In the fourth step, the case manager develops a *plan of action*. This process is one of organizing, securing, and integrating the necessary resources to meet the identified objectives and goals outlined in step four. The case plan may involve assistance in placing our client (Joe) within a residential, skilled, or nursing home facility in order to meet his current needs. With other cases, this may involve helping a client obtain necessary prescriptions or home health care, resolve transportation issues, or arrange home oxygen.

Whatever the identified need, the case manager documents the plan of action to meet the stated objectives/goals. Before proceeding to step five, collaborate with your patient to secure his or her understanding of the proposed plan. Include family members as applicable.

Coordinating services requires a case manager's expertise when *implementing the plan* necessary to meet the patient's identified needs. While executing the agreed plan of action, the case manager puts the pieces of the plan into motion. To successfully implement the stated plan, communication to all involved parties is once again vital.

Explain to your client the agencies available, and provide lists where applicable in every situation. Making the choice of facility or agency allows the parties to become actively involved in their own care planning. Also, the law mandates the patient's choice of agency.

Notify the agency or party who will contract or accept the patient's outlined plan to secure their services. Coordinate the onset of services and the delivery time or date, and keep the patient informed of all action plans. Follow up with a phone call to family members as indicated with the arrangement of services.

Remember when communicating with agencies to obtain contact names and fax numbers and give your own fax/phone number to ensure coordination of services. Also provide your client with a contact number so that he or she may reach you after hours with any concern or question that may arise. Communication is the cornerstone of implementing your plan of care to success.

Lastly, the sixth step is the case manager's *evaluation.* How effective were you as the case manager in reaching the desired objectives and goals? A case manager or any leader will tell you to always have an evaluation process in place to measure your success.

One idea worth mentioning is a patient follow-up call within twenty-four hours, again at three days, and repeated at seven days to inquire about the patient's satisfaction with the plan implementation. You may use conversation starters, such as "Were your meals delivered on time? Has the agency delivered your equipment? Do you understand your dismissal instructions?" If the client was discharged from a clinic, hospital, or a rehab setting, simply ask, "Do you understand your dismissal instructions?" Don't be afraid to ask if he or she has "Any questions?"

Another evaluation tool may simply be to mail a thank-you card that includes your business card for future reference. Make the time to simply write something like the following:

> Thank you, (patient name), for trusting me to
> coordinate your recent health-care needs. My goal
> is to provide you with the best service possible. I
> hope this service met with your satisfaction.
> Thanks again and best wishes,
> (Your name and credentials)
> Nurse Case Manager

Remember when completing the thank-you card to individualize the responses in accordance with the services arranged. Attaching your business card is easy and implies professionalism in your consulting skills. Many organizations are utilizing some form of written "thank-you" to clients served or mailing a survey for patients to provide feedback on services rendered.

Tip—*The* initial patient assessment *is the in-depth data collection process to identify the patient's needs in order to develop a comprehensive nursing case management plan. Once the initial assessment is completed, the case manager moves on to the next step, which is to* identify any real or potential needs. *Once you and your client agree on the problem or a need that requires your services, outline the* objectives and goals *for the process. In the fourth step, the case manager develops a* plan of action. *Coordinating services requires a case manager's expertise when* implementing the plan *necessary in order to meet the patient's identified needs. Lastly, the sixth step is the case manager's* evaluation.

Whether the evaluation process is in the form of a phone follow-up, a thank-you card, or a mailed survey to patients, please don't overlook this important case management process to closing out your nursing plan of care. Take the time to review your evaluation process and the feedback and look for new and creative ways to improve your case management skills.

The case manager who actively pursues an in-depth patient assessment, clues in to a perceived concern, identifies the patient need, outlines clear objectives and goals, issues a plan of action, executes the stated plan, and then evaluates the effectiveness of the plan will sharpen the skills necessary to become a successful case manager.

PATIENT PRESCRIPTION ASSESSMENT

As you become familiar with coordinating dismissal plans for patients, many common areas of need tend to surface among clients. The needs identified may include issues with transportation to and from appointments; coordinating outpatient services, such as therapies and infusions; and safety issues if a person lives alone.

In practicing case management, the nurse case manager will come in contact with a high number of clients who have issues with obtaining prescribed medications. This issue doesn't limit itself to only those individuals who have no insurance; it is becoming a common concern among many who are insured. You will hear that clients just don't have the co-payment to pick up the medication.

In efforts to seek alternative drug choices for the diagnosis, the client is informed that the drug prescribed is in accordance with practice recommendations for such a diagnosis.[5] Now, if you have been in health care for any length of time, you've no doubt run across ways to offset the costs encountered in obtaining the drugs prescribed.

The most logical approach is, of course, to check with your physician to see if a generic form of the drug exists. Generic forms are less expensive. People sometimes forget to ask because they think if the doctor prescribed it, they must need it. But what if this is the only drug prescribed and declared the only drug necessary to combat an infectious process, treat a specific heart condition, or manage a respiratory illness and known medical literature is supportive of this drug choice?

Whether your practice is within a hospital, clinic, health plan, or community setting, prescription assistance is becoming an increasingly common need. Therefore, let us quickly review the nursing process involved with prescription assistance (refer to Quick Reference Tools #8 and 9, Patient Prescription Assistance Guide and Patient Prescription Assistance Form) for further details.

As with the patient needs assessment, *the prescription assistance assessment* is in-depth data collection during the patient interview. Focus your efforts on the basics. What is the patient's residence? Obtain important contact information, such as a cell phone or evening telephone number. Inquire about and obtain the necessary information regarding the medical diagnosis that the prescribed

5. The Case Management Society of America, *CMAG Case Management Adherence Guidelines*, Version 2.0., (USA: Case Management Society of America, 2006).

drug is intended to help manage. Ask if any prior prescription services existed, which may include hospice services, home infusion needs, required injections, or gastrointestinal nutrition. Obtain the agencies involved with providing assistance.

Next, have the client identify any *prescription drug needs* they had during the hospital stay. Drug needs may also be identified during a physician appointment, outpatient visits to a clinic, or at an urgent care setting. Pay careful attention to what the families interpret as an identified drug need in light of financial commitments or any unusual social circumstances.

Sometimes, people won't divulge personal information or circumstances, as it may be embarrassing or they feel it is none of your business. A family member or friend may speak up on their behalf to make you aware of certain situations that may shed insight into possible avenues of prescription assistance.

Retrieve information related to the client's weekly, monthly, or yearly income status. The exact or estimated salary is important with attempts to obtain assistance through the many programs available. These programs may assist with delivery and coverage of medications prescribed to qualifying applicants.

Once he or she has reviewed all the information, the case manager pinpoints and collaborates with the client on an *identified drug or numerous prescription needs as stated*. Speak honestly with your client about the drug itself indicating its generic or brand names.

Sit down one-on-one to discuss the drug's impact with regard to the overall treatment as it relates to the client's illness or disease management. Answer any questions pertaining to the drug itself, and clarify with the physician as needed regarding unanswered issues. Always keep a current drug reference book handy in your personal library. The literature is a great resource for drug indications, actions, side effects, and usual dosing schedules pertaining to various methods of dispensing, such as oral, intravenous, topical, intramuscular, and subcutaneous.

This is a great opportunity for the nurse case manager to do some educating. Reinforce the drug's indication for treatment and why it is necessary to finish the prescribed amount. Encourage the client to stay the course, but remind him or her that if any untoward effects are noted to follow up with his or her physician for further guidance.

Provide any pamphlets, materials, or videos pertaining to the drug if applicable. Some institutions have prepared teaching sheets or video clips for certain drugs, which may be helpful in the education process. Allow plenty of time for questions and answers.

After the drug need is identified, the case manager will state the *objective or goal* in determining the process for prescription assistance. Individualize the objective/goal. The goal may be simply to "assist with obtaining home medications" or to "coordinate avenues for home medication assistance."

Insinuating you will "assist" or "coordinate" is not to indicate you will "obtain" in all cases the identified drug need for any client. The case manager's goal is to assist the client. As you will find in your practice of case management, not all medications are free.

Tip—*As the nurse case manager, you should be familiar with local, regional, state, and national programs that may help with prescription assistance. Keep a list of local pharmacies handy with important contact information for reference. Do your homework, and leave no base uncovered as you assist the client with the identified drug need.*

Sometimes, the plan of assistance is presented, and then the responsibility falls back on the client to follow through and pursue his or her own avenues or simply decline to take the medication. Yes, declining to take the prescribed medication is still the patient's right.

The case manager should go ahead and educate the client about the potential problems related to not following the recommendation of the physician. Be optimistic and realistic in setting the objectives and goals with the prescription assistance process.

The next step in this process is to develop a *plan of action.* As with the patient needs assessment guide, this step involves organizing and securing resources to help meet the identified goals/objectives.

Many avenues exist to help devise a successful plan to obtain the necessary drugs. Begin to look into available local competitive pricing markets for low-cost generic drugs. Grocery stores, as well as Walmart and similar shops, usually have comparable pricing with generic drugs. A low-cost drug for $4.00 to $5.00 helps all age groups.

Inquire to see if there is any personal means available to offset the cost of the drug, like a family trust fund, a bank CD, or credit cards. You won't know unless you ask. This goes back to client responsibility in an effort to abide by the recommended treatment plan.

Tap into your local nonprofit assistance programs designed to help those less fortunate access medical care. Some agencies also provide prescription assistance if the client meets eligibility requirements. As the case manager, you may have to help with filling out the application forms for pharmaceutical assistance programs.

As you assist with client needs, you will encounter many high-dollar drugs that patients simply can't afford. The pharmaceutical companies may have assistance programs available to those who meet the guidelines for free medication.[6]

Check into insurance prescription plans for guidance, and inquire about potential overrides or exceptions based on medical

---

6. U.S. Department of Health & Human Services, "Medicare 5 Ways to Lower Your Costs during the Coverage Gap," http://www.hhs.gov (accessed December 22, 2007).

necessity with attempts to lower patient co-pays. Ask the health plan if any disease management programs exist to help the client with management of their illness and with known prescription assistance processes.

As the nurse case manager, you should be familiar with local, regional, state, and national programs that may help with prescription assistance. Keep a list of local pharmacies handy for reference with important contact information. Do your homework, and leave no base uncovered as you assist the client with the identified drug need.

Once you've pursued the avenues available, begin the *implementation of the plan*. This is simply executing the plan utilizing the identified agencies that will be providing services to you and your client. Include the agency name, date of notification, and any contact information for documentation.

The execution of the plan is the part of the process in which you're closing in on the final preparations to secure the drugs to help your client. Touch base with all parties involved to fill in the communication gaps. Alert the patient and family or significant other involved with the planning process in order to get everyone on board.

Many are hanging by the phone awaiting the end results, hopeful a positive answer is coming their way. Review this step to ensure that you are meeting the outcomes you've identified during the process of objective/goal determination.

To conclude the case, you must have a method in place to *evaluate the plan* implemented in order to review your effectiveness as a case manager in securing your client's medications. This step may seem a little trivial, but it is necessary to complete the nursing process involved with any client.

Stick with the evaluation tools suggested earlier, such as following up by phone and mailing a thank-you card. For you, the case manager, these are simple methods to get you started. With practice, you may consider other alternatives, such as a home visit a few weeks later, brochure mailings, consulting services, or client surveys.

Patient-driven methods become the primary focus when following processes to ensure patient satisfaction. Not all cases will end satisfactorily, but knowing that you did everything possible to achieve the desired goals/objectives is a positive ending in itself.

Review any positive or negative comments received in a professional manner. Don't be hesitant to build upon your skills in order to make a successful career within the case management field. As a nurse case manager, you should stick with the basics of communication, individualize cases encountered, and ensure a timely follow-up with all clients. People appreciate honest efforts and will recognize those efforts in various ways. A simple "thank-you" is sometimes all we need to keep on keeping on.

You may need to reevaluate, redesign, or remarket your services at times to achieve your own goals/objectives.

CHAPTER 3

BALANCING UTILIZATION MANAGEMENT PRACTICE

In any field, new terms and abbreviations are part of the learning process. The nurse case manager's field is no exception. Many terms, ideas, concepts, and guidelines emerge, and as one starting out, one lacks this knowledge. What is utilization, and how does it fit into nursing case management practice? Don't fret. As you gain experience as a nurse case manager, you will begin to understand many facets in this new role.

As you will learn in the next chapter, the federal and state insurance programs of Medicare and Medicaid offer an extensive avenue for any case manager to pursue when assisting clients. A basic overview of each program will increase your knowledge base regarding these government programs. We covered care planning processes in the previous chapter and looked ahead to community resources and basic payer information. In addition, utilization management practice is also another area within the nurse case management field.

Utilization management is a major process of coordinating care. The nurse case manager coordinates the best care, at the best price, at the best level of entry, and with the collaboration of all parties to ensure the best quality of services. This process of utilization looks toward ensuring the medical necessity of admissions, the appropriate use of care levels as medically indicated, understanding of the approval days by the insurance review companies, and making certain that the patient is discharged from the hospital only when medically stable.[7] A few areas we will look at briefly in this chapter include the precertification process, insurance reviews, the denial process, length-of-stay issues, and hospital patient status.

Most utilization and case management programs also look into ways of decreasing hospital length-of-stay issues and tracking variance days, patient readmission rates, disease management, and favorable outcomes to improve upon the quality and delivery of patient care services. You, as the case manager, will begin to balance all these areas in order to achieve the desired goals determined by the leadership team of your facility.

PRECERTIFICATION PROCESS

Appropriate utilization practice begins in some of the following areas: the client's home, the physician's office, the outpatient clinic or unit of care, rehabilitation facilities, hospitals, nursing homes, and other areas of entry for delivery of health-care services.

A nurse case manager becomes involved to ensure proper steps are completed prior to certain procedures, tests, or even the admission of a client to an inpatient hospital or outpatient service area. This particular area of utilization is the precertification process.

As a nurse case manager, you may be responsible for pre-certifying the services recommended by a provider with the patient's insurance company. Some departments employ nurse reviewers to assist with this function as well as to perform clinical

---

7.   Mary Ann Huff, *Utilization Management Orientation* (Springfield, MO: St. Johns Mercy Hospital, 2010).

reviews as we will discuss later in this chapter. Secretarial or office staff can also be trained (according to facility guidelines) in this area of precertification.

Be prepared to wait with a telephonic precertification initiation. The insurance company's automatic phone system can be time-consuming to say the least. Just have the vital information, such as the client's birthday, policy number, and specifics as to demographics, handy when the customer service representative is available to chat one on one.

INSURANCE REVIEW

Utilization of services also encompasses the requested insurance clinical reviews. The payer may request reviews of those clients located in the hospital setting, skilled areas, or rehabilitation centers. As with any precertification process, the insurance may request clinical data to support the final decision of admission, continuing stay needs, or retrospectively, of care provided.

The decision to admit a patient to a facility for acute care needs is between the patient and his or her provider. But, as we know, insurance companies want the data to support a reason for acute care needs. The nurse case managers or utilization review nurses provide the initial information and continuing stay services needs based on several tools established by the utilization medical executive committee. This committee consists of a utilization medical director and administrative leadership.

The nurse case manager is the key liaison between the patient, the provider, and the payer.

A few reference tools, noted in circulation and updated annually, are the McKesson's Interqual Level of Care Criteria[8] and Milliman's Care Guidelines.[9] Just remember, these tools

8. McKesson Corporation, *McKesson InterQual Level of Care Criteria* (Newton, MA: McKesson Corporation, 2009).

9. Milliman Care Guidelines, "Delivering Evidence-based Knowledge at the Point of Care," http://www.careguidelines.com/ (accessed April 19, 2010).

are considered a practice guideline and collaboration with the physician may become necessary to obtain additional information to help with the certification process.

Continued service of your client's needs will also require a clinical review update provided to the insurance company as recommended. As you become familiar with providing the data required to support an admission and continuing stay based on the severity of the patient's illness and the intensity of service needs, you will begin to investigate the medical record for the specifics of the patient's condition rather quickly.

Regardless of the initial request, the insurance company inquires about the specifics of each client's case in order to certify those days of service. When in doubt, phone the insurance company and inquire as to the specifics in order to help with precertification of a recommended surgery, a simple procedure, home equipment needs, home care services, and even medication needs … just to name a few.

Always follow your established institutional policy regarding the clinical review format. Also refer to the Quick Reference Tool #6, which outlines a clinical review format and provides a sample review. The nurse case manager is wise to practice within established guidelines of practice in all areas and not just with clinical review formats in order to provide continuity of care to his or her clients.

It is much easier on the front end (while the patient is still in the facility) to provide the insurance with the requested information than to perform a retrospective review. This attention to providing the clinical review format accurately may indeed avert a future insurance denial.

DENIAL PROCESS

Let's look at the denial appeal claim process in short review. Most departments of case management and/or utilization have in place a process to address denials of claims. These appeal processes may include the nurse reviewer or a nurse case manager. Each follows those claims denied by the insurance company for payment of services delivered according to the contractual agreements. Consumers on the receiving end of health-care delivery also have rights to an appeal if their claims are denied. Our focus is on the nurse case manager's role in this process.

How do you know of a denial of a claim? The business office may alert the utilization staff of the denial, or your office may hear directly from the insurance, which is often the case, either by phone or received letter. By following the institutional guidelines for a denial of a claim, the nurse case manager or designee actively investigates the medical record to determine vital pieces of information that may have been overlooked in the initial and subsequent clinical data provided at an earlier time.

Communicating with the provider is essential in attempts to overturn the insurance company's initial denial of days or services. Most insurance companies offer a peer-to-peer review within the first days of the denial. Contact numbers provided help to ensure a live chat with a medical director of the health plan. After all, the insurance companies are just following their best customer service techniques to help diffuse a situation and keep it from enlarging.

It is easier on the front end to potentially prevent a denial than to overturn a denial with any argument about care. But in some cases, the patient receives the denial letter and thus begins the investigation of the medical record. Clinical review nurses and nurse case managers become the investigators of the medical record.

Why investigate? Because you, the nurse case manager, have the knowledge of disease processes and practice guidelines that enables you to look for key parts of care provided. These key elements of care provided help substantiate the delivery of care that was essential to the client's needs at the time of service. In addition, this investigation of the medical record is a unique task to the investigator.

Make no mistake about the one investigating the case. This is the "go-to" person when someone needs to know how to do the right thing in nursing case management practices. This person is actively involved in the pursuit of making the department run smoothly. He or she is a high achiever, self-motivated, is involved in the committee, has the latest tools in the trade, and is loaded with a wealth of knowledge. You, as the new employee in the department of case management or utilization, may be thinking of a person in your office who may indeed fit this profile.

The denial appeal process includes the investigation of the medical record to pull information that may support the claim submitted. It may provide clues to enhance your practice techniques with future cases. Communicating with the provider involved with the case may also add additional information quite possibly not known previously.

Encourage the parties (insurance medical director and physician) to connect early in helping with clarification of the case in question. If the peer-to-peer communication is lacking, utilize established forms to allow the provider to have his or her turn to explain the treatment details. But realistically, it may be harder than you think to get action elicited, as physicians are also extremely busy.

Be willing to offer any suggestions that could possibly help to certify the care rendered, such as abnormal labs, test results, continued intravenous medication needs, or even the explanation as to the delay in a possible procedure related to the instability of the client's condition. Whatever the potential scenario you're tasked with trying to overturn during the appeal process, remember to offer your assistance willingly in an attempt to cushion the message conveyed. Your positive efforts will enhance your future connections when similar appeals/denials occur.

LENGTH-OF-STAY ISSUES

Another component of utilization practice involves length-of-stay (LOS) issues. With any admission to an acute care facility, a suspected diagnosis is determined. Once the diagnosis is determined, based on information provided by the patient or a family member, the physician begins a workup. This workup usually includes an established battery of lab tests, x-rays, assessment of the client's systems, and procedures to help determine a primary diagnosis or problem list that necessitates a treatment plan. The treatment plan is vital to the patient's recovery or cure or the stabilization of symptoms if the client's prognosis is poor.

During this time of evaluation and treatment, the aim is to help the client return to a baseline of functional capacity in order to return home or in some cases, to alternative levels of care. Practice guidelines established by the institution's utilization medical executive committee help to guide the nurse case manager according to the client's severity of illness and intensity of service needs. In reviewing these guidelines, you will also be expected to ascertain, by established criteria, when a client might be ready for dismissal from the acute care setting.

Visual contact with the client assessment helps you determine anticipated dismissal needs. After all, the case manager is to help coordinate the client's care with appropriate utilization of resources necessary to meet the desired patient outcomes.

A large part of case management is looking at the average length of stay related to the client's diagnosis and helping the client toward a dismissal plan once medically stable enough to leave the acute care setting. This is a true balancing act for case managers. Why? Because, you're balancing the medical stability and the continued stay needs of your client to ensure the appropriate utilization of care. Utilization and case management both provide the patient with the "right care, at the right time, and in the right place."[10]

I finally said it, *the right place.* In order to be good stewards of utilization, nurse case managers inquire about continued treatment plans when care may be provided at an alternative level, such as the patient's home. Length-of-stay issues *not* based on medical necessity become a bigger issue if not addressed.

Tip—*A few common red flags to any nurse case manager tracking length-of-stay issues are social issues, lack of transportation, medication needs, and late physician rounding.*

In tracking length-of-stay issues, your facility usually has established tracking mechanisms intact for the nurse case manager to assist with data collection. You will quickly learn the issues that surround increased length-of-stay problems as you become familiar with your role. A few common red flags to any nurse case manager tracking length-of-stay issues are social issues, lack of transportation, medication needs, and late physician rounding.

Other items of concern include system issues, coordination of outside services in a timely fashion, guardianship or family dynamics, and the availability/acceptance of outlying facilities to meet the client's needs upon dismissal. Variance days contribute to increased length of stay and increase health claim costs. Failure to perform a needed procedure because of equipment failure, scheduling delays, or possibly a twenty-four/seven operational issue can drive up costs and tack on unnecessary days.

The nurse case manager's knowledge of disease processes and treatment guidelines helps to identify the variance days. By tracking these days, he or she obtains a wealth of information. The information gathered will assist the business office and administrators of any facility to identify areas that may need

10.   Mary Ann Huff, *Case Management Orientation, UR, UM and CM: The Basics* (Springfield, MO: St John's Mercy Hospital, 2005).

improvement for the delivery of care in a timely and cost-effective manner.

Whatever database your facility chooses to track the variance days that may drive up health-care costs, the nurse case manager is in a position to identify the cause and quite possibly interact to help avoid future delays by being on the front line. Of course, the system issues need the attention and directive of administrators to correct.

Communication and professional collaboration with the health-care team, providers, and, most important, the client is essential. You should communicate early in the admission of the client to a hospital setting or clinic with the client's nurse and the physician or designee.

As you review the medical record, look for clues to patient stability in order to formulate and coordinate a safe dismissal plan. Also look into any possible barriers to the treatment plan or dismissal plan, and facilitate where possible a safe dismissal plan for the client. Communicating with all parties is crucial during the assessment, planning, delivery, and evaluation of care.

HOSPITAL PATIENT STATUS

We will end this chapter with a discussion of patient admission types. The correct patient status of hospitalized clients assists the business office to ensure appropriate billing of charges. It is necessary to determine the appropriate status assigned with the delivery of care, such as outpatient, observation, or inpatient status types. Employees identified to assist with this process include nurse case managers, nurse reviewers, nursing staff, secretarial staff, admission representatives, billing coders, and providers.

The provider usually determines the patient admission status type with the initial orders. Many facilities use an electronic medical record and have implemented order sets or prompts to guide the provider with the appropriate selection. Guidelines and updates in identifying appropriate status types is communicated to providers by the insurance companies, Medicare, Medicaid, and hospital administrators.

Correcting the admission type is essential and time sensitive early on in the admission of a client for services and before dismissal according to mandated guidelines by the contracted health plans. Why involve the nurse case managers? This process is delegated to frontline individuals who routinely review medical records. The emergency department is the area in which to look first in determining if the documentation supports an inpatient admission.[11] Nurse case managers use admission criteria guidelines in review of the medical record, and the patient status types are referenced in these guidelines.

Outpatient status types indicate those patient services best served in an outpatient setting or clinic. Health insurance plans provide a list of outpatient procedures that are billed to insurance companies. This approved list may be grouped into specialty areas, such as cardiac, cardiothoracic, gastrointestinal, and surgery to name a few.

A client may be listed as an observation or inpatient admission with your facility upon the initial review of the record. The provider may in error select the wrong status type when inputting orders. One of the first people to look for in case management will be the case manager to ascertain the attending provider's orders for status type.

In doing so, you will use established guidelines to determine if the status type is appropriate to the diagnosis, presenting signs and symptoms, and treatment plan outlined. Sometimes the documentation doesn't support the patient status type, and therefore the case manager needs to follow up with the physician for discussion. In this instance, the case manager acts as a conduit of information for the physician and helps him or her assign the

---

11.   D. Hale and K. A. Bower, "Observation or Inpatient? Correct Patient Status More Critical than Ever," *Hospital Case Management* 16(6) (2008), 81–84.

correct status to the patient. This benefits the patient, provider, and payer of care.

Communication with the provider may be necessary to help in determining the diagnosis, plan of treatment, and appropriate patient status type. If these items are not readily available for review in the medical record, a need for clarification exists. This provides an opportunity for the provider to update the medical record to reflect his or her intentions with the care plan.

This chapter deals with a few topics related to utilization management that involve the nurse case manager. Utilization becomes to the seasoned nurse case manager a balancing of practice between utilization and case management functions. Depending on the caseload, dismissal plans, and insurance requests, the nurse case manager uses time management and prioritization to best manage cases.

As with any new role, stress levels may be high while you are learning about it and its processes. Remember to apply your best customer skills and always use effective communication styles to accommodate all parties involved to achieve the maximally desired outcomes. Put on your best grin and bear it. It's a cheesy phrase, I know, but it's effective when situations have a tendency to spin out of control.

Tip—*Utilization becomes to the seasoned nurse case manager a balancing of practice between utilization and case management functions. Depending on the caseload, dismissal plans, and insurance requests, the nurse case manager uses time management and prioritization to best manage cases.*

The nurse case manager uses the established utilization plan guidelines in reviewing the medical record to help to determine the appropriate patient status type. Consult the utilization plan medical director for clarification and guidance. As a nurse case manager, always follow the institutional processes with any identified problem areas in need of correction.

Chapter 4

Medicare and Medicaid

Medicare and Medicaid were created during President Lyndon Johnson's presidency. This health-care option provided insurance to qualifying elderly and disabled persons and provided medical assistance to low-income persons. Both programs are federally financed. In addition to federal funds, Medicaid insurance also receives state financing.[12]

In this chapter, we will look into information basics regarding the federally funded programs of Medicare and Medicaid. Following are specific Web links to further investigate the programs, as well as information for client assistance.

Medicare Basics

The Medicare insurance is provided for people age sixty-five or older, qualifying disabled parties, and anyone with kidney failure. The Web sites for this program are www.cms.hhs.gov or www.medicare.gov. These sites provide additional in-depth information for review. They are updated frequently for consumers (see also

---

12. S. Daniels and M. Ramey, *The Leader's Guide to Hospital Case Management* (Sudbury, MA: Jones and Bartlett Publishers, 2005).

Quick Reference Tool #1 for further Medicare information basics).

Medicare provides basic coverage of health-care costs. Unfortunately, not all medical expenses are paid. The traditional Medicare insurance has two parts, Part A and Part B. An eligible person has the option of choosing the traditional Medicare Part A and B plans or may elect to have a Medicare Advantage Plan or Part C. Part C plans include the following: a health maintenance organization (HMO), a preferred provider organization (PPO), and a provider sponsored organization (PSO).

As mentioned, not all costs are covered, as with most insurance plans. Therefore, many private insurance companies sell Medi-gap or supplemental insurance to help with deductibles, coinsurance, prescription drugs, and possible services not covered by Medicare. Additionally, prescription Part D plans exist to help with medication needs.[13]

The eligible party must review all possible insurance options with Medicare and determine the best possible plan that fits their lifestyle, budget, and anticipated future needs. These insurance options can be somewhat confusing. Any questions should be directed to your local Social Security office. You can also call 1-800-772-1213 or visit this Web site: www.socialsecurity.gov.

You may also refer to www.medicare.gov or www.hhs.gov for additional information and guidance.

As a nurse case manager, it is vital you have a basic understanding of the Medicare insurance plan. More likely than not, your largest client pool will be utilizing a traditional Medicare Part A and B with a supplemental Medi-gap plan or opting to have one of the Part C Medicare Advantage Plans. Patients and their families may come to you with questions or problems associated with their Medicare plans.

It may at times be difficult for anyone to know for certain if the insurance selected is the best option for his or her needs.

---

13. The National Underwriter Company, *Tax Facts 2006 All About Medicare* (Cincinnati, OH: The National Underwriter Company, 2006).

With that said, sometimes, a consumer doesn't know if he or she has a good car or home insurance plan until a claim is submitted. Only once the claims are reviewed and processed can we begin to understand the coverage we've purchased. At that moment, we actually begin to see what type of service we have. Then, pending the customer flexibility or inflexibility, we may shop around for a better deal.

TIP—*The nurse case manager who continues to update his or her files and knowledge base with the latest information regarding Medicare insurance is one step ahead in caseload planning.*

Likewise, the eligible Medicare client may have initially selected a plan, but he or she may not know how well the plan reimburses until the claims are submitted. As the nurse case manager and patient advocate, you can encourage the patient or family member to notify the insurance plan to obtain answers to questions regarding benefits, reimbursement, coinsurance, etc.

Guide the patient/family with a set of prepared questions to have ready when a member representative contact is made. Being prepared will help keep the conversation on track and elicit answers to the questions needed for the patient's satisfaction.

Questions to have the client ask the insurance company may simply be something like: Do I have to pay any deductibles with a hospital admission? What specific benefits entitle me to skilled care at home or within a nursing facility? What is my total out-of-pocket maximum cost? Encourage the client to ask for the details of the insurance plan in writing to avoid future problems.

MEDICAID BASICS

Another avenue to medical care is with the Medicaid program. This insurance is provided by each state with its own set of rules regarding the implementation of the program. Many groups benefit with the available medical care at no cost based on each state's program.[14] The Quick Reference Tool #2 highlights important information pertaining to Medicaid recipients.

You should tap into the state's Web site to find the Medicaid criteria in order to better serve clients in your immediate service area. Please refer to www.cms.hhs.gov to obtain additional information regarding this government program.

The Medicaid program assists, as mentioned, the many groups of individuals who might not have any other means available to receive health care. Some groups who might be eligible to receive this program include low-income families, children, the elderly, disabled persons, and pregnant women. Most are truly thankful to have the opportunity to have their health-care needs met.

The nurse case manager who continues to update his or her files and knowledge base with the latest information regarding Medicare insurance is one step ahead in caseload planning. Please attach a bookmark to www.medicare.gov on your personal computer, and refer to it at least quarterly for additional updates to the Medicare program as outlined by the government. With colleague collaboration and networking, keep your ears and eyes open to any additional information that may impact your current nursing case management practice.

An informed case manager is a wise patient advocate, while always striving to stay ahead of the constant changes within the case management field.

14. U.S. Department of Health & Human Services, "Centers for Medicare & Medicaid Services," http://www.hhs.gov (accessed December 22, 2007).

CHAPTER 5

TAPPING INTO COMMUNITY RESOURCES

So far, we've learned a few basics of case management, utilization practice, the case manager role, Medicare, Medicaid, and related important tips. We've discussed the nursing process as it applies to patient assistance and prescription needs. Now what? Where does a case manager find the resources necessary to tackle the caseload needs?

Where do I look to find the local, regional, and even state assistance to help guide my patients? Do I begin with Web surfing, local government agencies, or the yellow pages? Information is available at your fingertips if you know where to begin the search.

DEVELOP A COMMUNITY DATABASE

First of all, begin a database and label it "Community Resources." Accomplish this small task by creating an electronic document with agency names and contact numbers, a Rolodex card system, or even a file system. I prefer to use all three avenues and also utilize a backup disc.

As a nurse case manager, first and foremost, look into what your community has to offer, and branch out from there to regional, state, and federal program agencies in building your files. As you begin networking with vendors, case managers, social workers, government representatives, and other allied health professionals, the information will pour in, and before you know it, you have a database at your fingertips.

Community resources may be obvious to some nurse case managers, but they can be a struggle to obtain for those starting out in the role. A few areas to begin the search include the following:

> **Medical alert services**—Help clients live independently at home by utilizing a personal response system for emergency services.

> **Local departments of aging**—These agencies help to plan, develop, and fund projects that enhance the quality of life of older adults. Many include services at senior centers, transportation assistance, meal programs, and information with in-home assistance.

> **Home health agencies**—Offer in-home services with nursing, personal care, therapists, and monitoring equipment that provides important daily information regarding a client's condition. Services are aimed at helping a client to recover from an injury or illness and providing postoperative care and instruction/education as indicated, while helping the client to remain independent.

> **Transportation services**—Services aimed at providing transportation for in-home clients, hospital transports to other facilities, transport

for clients returning home, and transport in unusual circumstances.

Rehabilitation centers—Centers that provide care and treatment for a variety of clients by highly trained specialists. These centers focus on helping clients with regaining strength, cognition, communication, and motor skills damaged by stroke or brain injury, ventilator weaning, and complex medical needs.

Personal care services—A variety of services to assist clients in home with meal preparation, transportation, housekeeping, bathing and grooming, shopping, and transfer assistance in and out of bed.

Home parenteral services—Trained professionals who assist with home intravenous needs. They provide assistance in home while maintaining quality of life, reducing risk of infections, and with less cost than with a hospital stay.

Medical equipment agencies—Provide client equipment needs, which include but are not limited to oxygen supplies, wheelchairs, hospital beds, bedside commodes, walkers, mattresses, trapeze bars, ambulatory supplies, nutrition, wound and dressing applications, and specialty application devices for home or vehicles.

Outpatient clinic services—Services aimed at assisting the client who is not homebound to receive intravenous antibiotic therapy, blood transfusion products, special intravenous medications, hydration therapy, and cardiac treatments aimed at enhancement of heart function.

Division of Family Services—Department of social services that provides assistance to families.

Day-care facilities—Facilities that offer daytime health services to give relief to caregivers of clients with disabilities or chronic illnesses.

In addition to the above, other agencies to investigate, which may help broaden your search, include nursing homes, assisted-living facilities, Medicare skilled facilities, counseling service agencies, support groups, legal aid assistance, state Medicare and Medicaid numbers, divisions of social services, area councils of churches, senior citizens' offices, housing assistance and shelters, food banks, free clinic care agencies, and free medication clinics. This is just the beginning of a list. As your practice and experience enlarges, so will your filing system of available agencies and services.

Tip—*As a nurse case manager, first and foremost, look into what your community has to offer and branch out from there to regional, state, and federal program agencies in building your files.*

When devising a plan of action for your specific client needs, encourage agency choices from a list that you provide for client review. Agency choice is best when made by your client, as it relieves you of promoting one agency over another. It also allows the client to become an active participant in planning his or her health-care needs.

Allowing the client to become an active participant in meeting his or her own care needs is important in building trust in the nurse case manager's efforts and responsibility for his or her own health. At times though, the nurse case manager coordinates services by contacting a designated family member or significant other who is looking out for the client's best interest.

As a case manager involved with arrangement of services, inquire with insurance companies about the recommended in-network providers. Provide this information to the client, and if needed, on behalf of the client, clarify insurance benefits for certain services, such as equipment costs and co-pays.

Remember to update your filing system as your contacts and knowledge of area services enlarge. Organization is essential to time management in your practice as a nurse case manager.

CHAPTER 6

QUICK REFERENCE TOOLS

How do you begin to filter through processes and implement a plan of care as a nurse case manager? Policies in the corporate world revolve around a certain step process to help clarify and guide employers and employees in facility operations. These operations in most employer groups may include job benefits, time off, employee do's and don'ts, and grievances polices.

Under health-care operations specific to satisfactory patient care outcomes, one might utilize processes devoted to patient care satisfaction, disease management, billing practices, obtaining authorizations, denials and appeals, and most important, processes that affect the day-to-day care of an individual. You'll notice there are books devoted to policies of all sorts on the shelves and information available via the Internet.

If you're like most staff, you want the important pieces of data necessary to perform your job duties readily available at your fingertips. You also want that information quickly, sparing you every available minute in your already complicated day. Time is of the essence when assessing, devising, and initiating a client's plan of care. After all, it's easier to follow a few steps than a three-page algorithm in arranging a particular service for a client.

Information specific to formulating a plan of care is essential in having some type of organizational process as a nurse case manager. What? We have to be organized? Many a person will argue that outward appearances are deceiving and that a cluttered desk equates with a genius at work. So develop the organizational method that works best for you.

One important aspect related to coordinating services is the patient's agreement with using your expertise in handling these arrangements—in other words, a patient contracts for the case management services.

This particular tool is probably the most important in establishing up front your intentions on the person's behalf. The content addresses the written agreement or contract between you and the client. Securing your professional services is practical and required in some instances.

You may want to check with your employer if such a document is necessary prior to serving the clients in your area of practice. Case management services may be a service provided for free, according to certain health plan groups, hospitals, or health systems. Independent case managers utilize some written agreement in order to coordinate case management services. You may want to consult an attorney in order to formulate your own consent form.

Remember that this tool, as well as the others to follow, is only meant as a guide to enhance your practice.

Having the concise information available at your fingertips will only help to manage your time effectively as a case manager, and let's face it; you want to save valuable time with your cases. Who wants to spend several hours going through files to only come up empty-handed?

As the day evolves, any tool to make your job easier becomes a must. The following tools may be helpful in streamlining your processes. Keep these quick reference tools handy.

TOOL #1: MEDICARE INFORMATION TOOL—2010

Medicare Part A: the Basics

> Hospital deductible Part A = 1–60 days (co-pay applies), 61–90 days (co-pay applies), and 91–150 days (co-pay applies). The benefit period is sixty days. Part A benefits cover inpatient hospital care, hospice, home health, and skilled facility care. The patient is responsible for costs accumulated after more than 150 days.

Medicare Part B: the Basics

> Part B deductible applies. The benefit coverage is for physician visits and services, outpatient care, physical therapy, medical equipment, and ambulance services.

Quick Notes:

1. Coverage is 100 percent for home health-care services if a patient is homebound.
2. The patient can choose any Medicare certified home health agency.
3. Homemaker services are not covered by Medicare.
4. Coverage is 80 percent for qualified medical equipment and 20 percent coinsurance.
5. Skilled nursing facility coverage is 100 percent for one to twenty days if eligible, and coinsurance is applicable for Medicare in days twenty-one to one hundred. If the care need requires greater than one hundred days, then the care continues or other options are exhausted with discussions regarding patient financial responsibility revisited.
6. Uses Medicare guidelines for services with no authorization usually required. If it is a Medicare HMO plan, then verify benefits with the health plan.

7. Check with the supplemental insurances if the client has skilled facility coinsurance coverage.
8. If the Medicare number ends with a letter *M*, then this indicates the patient only has Part B coverage and the secondary insurance may expect precertification for services.
9. Check with Medicare HMO/PPO plans to determine the coinsurance coverage. Verify benefits for home health care, skilled facility, and home equipment as the plan may differ from traditional Medicare benefits.

Please refer to www.medicare.gov for information on further benefits of this program.

TOOL #2: MEDICAID INFORMATION TOOL—2010

Medicaid is a medical assistance program funded by the state and federal governments for American families of low-income status and assistive services. Each state's applicants must meet the state's own eligibility standards. Eligibility in one state doesn't necessarily mean eligibility in another; the same requirements may not exist in another state. Medicaid also provides a supplement to Medicare insurance coverage. If a person qualifies, Medicaid will pay the Medicare premium, coinsurances, and deductibles.

Quick Notes:
1. Coverage allowed for extended nursing home care
2. Coverage for inpatient hospital and outpatient services
3. Coverage for prenatal care
4. Coverage for children's vaccinations
5. Coverage for physician services
6. Coverage for home health care skilled nursing visits

7. Coverage for lab and x-rays
8. Coverage for rural health clinic services
9. Coverage for prescription drug assistance

Please refer to www.cms.hhs.gov/MedicaidGenInfo/ for further information on the benefits of this program.

TOOL #3: CASE MANAGEMENT PATIENT NEEDS ASSESSMENT GUIDE

1. Patient assessment—The process of in-depth data collection to identify real or potential patient needs in order to develop a comprehensive case management plan. Data include:
   - Demographics
   - Medical diagnosis (current and past)
   - Current living arrangements
   - Self-care deficits
   - Advance directives
   - Financial issues, etc.
   - Prior services and agency support
2. Patient/family perceived or voiced concerns
3. Case manager–identified patient needs based on above information
4. Case manager objective and goals—An outlined statement of the identified problem and/or need with an individualized outlined objective and goal
5. Case manager plan of action—The process of organizing, securing, and integrating resources necessary to meet the identified objective and goal
6. Case manager implementation of plan—The execution of the above plan of action to assist in accomplishment of stated objective and goals

7. Case manager evaluation of plan—To determine the case management plan effectiveness in reaching the desired objective and goals

TOOL #4: PATIENT ASSESSMENT FORM

1. Referral Date:
2. Name: (address) City State Zip code Home/Cell Phone # Emergency Contact Relation/Phone/Cell # Employer/Phone # Primary Care Physician Other Physician Consults Date of Birth Age Sex Race
3. Insurance: Insurance Identification # Other Insurance and Identification #
4. Medical History/Diagnosis:

5. Data Collection (circle):
Lives alone? Yes/No
If no, explain:
Advance Directive? Yes/No
Self-care? Yes/No
If no, explain:
Financial Issues? Medications? Equipment?
Expect change? Yes/No
If yes, explain:
Home caregiver? Yes/No
Nursing home resident/assisted living/group home
Facility name:
Homeless/shelter/long-term facility
Facility name:

6. Prior Services (circle)
Home health care/home infusion/hospice/medical equipment/Meals on Wheels/
intravenous nutrition/tube feedings/homemakers/personal services
Agency Name:
Agency Name:
Agency Name:

7. Patient/Family Perceived or Voiced Concern:

8. Case Manager Identified Patient Need:

9. Case Manager Objective/Goal:

10. Case Manager Plan of Action:

11. Case Manager Implementation of Plan:
Agency notified (date):
Phone #:
Fax #:
Agency notified (date):
Phone #:
Fax #:

12. Case Manager Evaluation of Plan:
Phone follow-up call (date):
Phone follow-up call (date):
Case closed (date):
Mail thank-you card (date):

TOOL #5: RESOURCE LIST

The following resources are just the beginning in your efforts to comb the Web for vital information to assist your clients. By now, you realize that many avenues exist. Anyone can update his or her knowledge base using these connections. It's as easy as 1-2-3.

As you begin to build upon your practice, take advantage of these sites and be sure to compile your own list as you network. Familiarize yourself with local agency Web sites and government office links to round out the connections.

Many clients and co-workers will benefit from any information you obtain in efforts with medication assistance, finding a reputable nursing home, care of the elderly, and many other health-care agencies. Armed with this tool, the case manager finds the answers needed while helping others. You will access these sites frequently for any updates to their services. Frequently throughout the year, updates are posted to ensure that the public is informed of upcoming changes, events, and new laws affecting the site's services.

> www.medicare.gov (Medicare)
> www.CMS.gov (Center for Medicare and Medicaid)
> www.officeofaging.com
> www.mealsonwheels.com
> www.eldercarelink.com
> www.needymeds.com
> www.prescriptionassistance.com
> www.wal-mart.com (Resource for low-cost medications)
> www.k-mart.com (Resource for low-cost medications)
> www.nursinghomes.com
> www.medicalequipment.com
> www.rehabilitationcare.com

www.cms.hhs.gov.com
www.ccmcertification.gov/ (the case manager certification Web site)
www.socialsecurity.gov
www.nachc.com (National Association of Community Health Centers)
www.narhc.org (National Association of Rural Health Clinics)
www.hhs.gov/fbci (The faith-based community programs)
www.CovertheUninsured.org
www.govbenefits.gov (The official benefits Web site)
www.insurekids.gov- (A free or low-cost health insurance for qualifying families)

Tool #6: Clinical Review Format

As mentioned in chapter 3, insurance or review companies request clinical information related to a hospital admission by either a nurse case manager or a utilization review nurse. This information is vital in helping with certification of an admission or a continued stay while the patient is hospitalized.

Policies should be in place to provide only information pertinent to the hospital admission in order to protect privacy requirements of patients. Many companies utilize an approved program or template when providing clinical data to the insurance company.

The following basic format is useful when reviewing the information located in the electronic record or the patient chart. The necessary information can be retrieved utilizing a systematic approach with each case review.

Case managers following this organizational method outlined below will find the process efficient and effective for obtaining authorization from the insurance or review companies. If no method exists, the resulting random collection of information may elicit numerous phone calls from the review or insurance company and possibly result in a denial of days requested.

- Diagnosis or current problem stated
- History documented
- Procedures/dates
- Current date and time
- Follow dated entry with specifics such as vital signs, assessment findings, complaints, x-rays, lab work, medications given
- Treatment plan
- Request certification days with expected clinical review future date
- End note with your initials or according to facility policy

SAMPLE CLINICAL REVIEW

ADMISSION MEDICAL REVIEW

Diagnosis: Acute myocardial infarction
History: CABG 2008, Hypertension, Diabetes
Procedure: Emergent heart angiogram with stent to the LAD (left ascending diagonal branch) 11/10/08
On 11/11/2010 13:00, Patient admitted 11/11 through the emergency room with complaints of chest pain. The duration of pain is three hours prior to arrival. An EKG revealed ST elevation in leads 2, 3, AVF and V2–V4. Lab work as follows: troponin level 20, complete blood count normal, basic metabolic profile is normal. Given intravenous morphine, intravenous nitroglycerin, intravenous aggrastat, intravenous heparin,

sublingual nitroglycerin given x3, aspirin 325 mg given x1. The patient was then taken to the heart catherization lab emergently and found with a 100 percent left ascending diagonal occlusion. Stented lesion to 0 percent residual status. **Treatment plan:** Intensive care unit postoperatively and begin Plavix 75 mg daily, aspirin 325 mg daily, continue intravenous aggrastat until bag infuses, begin metoprolol 25 mg twice a day, lisinopril 5 mg twice a day, low cholesterol diet, cardiac rehab education, bed rest 6 hours and begin activity.

On 11/12/2010 9:00 AM, no pain. Vital signs stable. Ambulating. Troponin level peaked at 30.1. The patient is tolerating medications. **Treatment plan**: Discharge home, follow-up two weeks with primary care physician, and a one-month follow-up with cardiology. Please certify the stay with an update expected 11/14/2010. (your initials or name)

(Institutional logo, disclaimer information)

TOOL #7: PAYER BASICS

The information which is given and signed by the patient for treatment should include a written statement that your company or facility will communicate with insurance carriers regarding claims and care provided. If no statement exists, the nurse case manager must ask permission and document such permission in order to contact the insurance carrier.

Once the information is collected regarding insurance name and policy number, the nurse case manager or designee (clerical staff) will notify the insurance of the patient's admission to the hospital setting. Regardless of inpatient or outpatient services, nurse case managers should check with the patient's insurance regarding benefits for service, determine if any prior precertification is required, and then arrange those services.

When calling insurance companies, there are a few pieces of information you will need in order to navigate quickly through automatic lines or in conversation with a member representative. Be prepared to give the reason for the inquiry regarding services, such as inpatient hospital admission, outpatient services, home health, medical equipment, in-home caregivers, skilled facility plans, acute rehab transitional care, and therapy needs, which may include speech, physical, and occupational assistance. The following information should be readily available when asking for precertification or benefits on the client's behalf.

- Patient name
- Provider and Tax ID
- Provider address
- Provider contact number
- Birthday
- Address
- Policy number
- Employer group
- Service requested

To clarify benefit information for a particular service requested, the following information is useful to any nurse case manager when developing a patient care plan. Consider the insurance plan benefit and any potential costs incurred by the patient.

- In-network coverage
- Out-of-network coverage
- Co-pays
- Deductibles
- Out-of-pocket maximum dollars as applicable to the case

- Allowable skilled facility days per benefit period or year
- Allowable visits per calendar year for home health care and therapy needs

Remember to always try to reach a member representative if any questions exist following the automatic responses obtained. Ideally, speaking with a live person will save you time. The automatic recorded systems lack information pieces vital to a case manager's inquiries and unfortunately hinder our work flow and ability to manage cases efficiently.

Share benefit information obtained with the client when arranging services and also encourage the patient to call his or her insurance carrier if any questions surface. Most patients are grateful for any assistance, as they too find it difficult to navigate the automatic systems.

Finally, the nurse case manager should document important information received in a secure case file. Please follow your institutional polices to ensure privacy guidelines are being followed and to avoid legal repercussions. For those who are nurse case manager entrepreneurs of case management businesses, obtain legal guidance in adherence to local, state, and federal privacy regulations.

Tool #8: Patient Prescription Assistance Guide

Patient assessment—The process of in-depth data collection to identify real or potential patient prescription needs in order to develop a comprehensive case management plan.

- Demographics
- Medical diagnosis (current/past)
- Financial issues, insurance, social issues that may affect ability to obtain medications prescribed

- Prior prescription service
- Patient and/or family perceived voiced prescription drug need
- Case manager–identified prescription drug needs based on above information
- Current drug information from reference book
- List of usual drug costs
- Drug education information sheets

Case manager objective and goal—An outlined statement of the identified problem or need with an individualized outlined objective and goal.

Case manager plan of action—The process of organizing, securing, and integrating resources necessary to the identified objective and goal.

- Local pharmacy lists
- Local agency assistance programs
- Local participating pharmacy discount medication lists

Case manager implementation of plan—The execution of the above plan of action to assist with accomplishment of the stated objective and goal and communication of plans arranged with patient, family, or significant other.

Case manager evaluation of plan—To determine the case management plan effectiveness in reaching the desired objective and goals.

- Phone follow-up within twenty-four hours
- Future problems in securing prescribed medications
- Mail thank-you card and include business card

TOOL #9: PATIENT PRESCRIPTION ASSISTANCE FORM

1. Referral date:
2. Name: Primary care physician: Office contact #: Other physician consults: Office contact #: Patient address: City State Zip code Phone/cell # Emergency contact: Relation/phone/cell # Employer/phone #
3. Insurance: Insurance identification # Other insurance identification #
4. Medical History/Diagnosis:
5. Data Collection (circle): Live alone? Yes/No If no, explain: Financial issues? Medications? Equipment? Self-care? Yes/No If no, explain: Weekly income $ Monthly income $ Yearly income $ Expect change: Yes/No If yes, explain: Home caregiver? Yes/No Nursing home resident/assisted living/group home Facility name: Homeless/shelter/long-term care facility Facility name:

6. Prior Prescription Services (circle):
Hospice/medical equipment/intravenous nutrition/tube feedings/home infusion/other
Assistive programs? Yes/No
Agency name:
Agency name:
Agency name:

7. Patient/Family Perceived or Voiced Prescription Concern:

8. Case Manager Identified Patient Prescription Need:
Drug name:
Education:

9. Case Manager Objective/Goal:

10. Case Manager Plan of Action:
Pharmacies/generic or low-cost drugs:
Pharmaceutical assistance programs/forms:
Charity application forms:
Legal assistance programs:
Credit card (circle): Yes/No
Insurance disease management assistance:
Pharmacy payment plans:
Outpatient services (short supply of drugs):

11. Case Manager Implementation of Plan:
Agency notified (date):
Phone #
Fax #
Agency notified (date):
Phone #
Fax #
Patient and family notified (date):

12. Case Manager Evaluation of Plan:
Phone follow-up call (date):
Phone follow-up call (date):
Case closed (date):
Mail thank-you card (date):

TOOL #10: CONSENT FOR CASE MANAGEMENT SERVICES

This tool is probably the most important. It addresses the written contract between you and the client. Securing your professional services is practical and required in some instances. In your communications with your client, he or she must be made aware of their patient rights in keeping with the health insurance portability act.[15] Most facilities have a basic statement pertaining to patient rights, and a copy is offered to patients and/or families upon contact with any provider.

The case management contract between the case manager and client is also a useful tool in securing services. You may want to check with your employer if such a document is necessary prior to your serving the clients in your area of practice. The consent authorizes the nurse case manager to obtain information relative to the patient's condition and to communicate with providers and payers and allows for the case management services.[16]

Remember that this tool, as well as the others listed previously, is only a guide to enhance your practice. You may want to consult a legal professional to formulate your own form.

SAMPLE CONTRACT

Consent for Case Management

Patient name:
I acknowledge receiving written information explaining the nurse case manager's role with case management services. I understand the nurse case manager will work with me and the health-

---

15. C. M. Mullahy and D. K. Jensen, *Student Study Guide to Accompany The Case Manager's Handbook*, 3rd ed. (Sudbury, MA: Jones and Bartlett, 2004).
16. Ibid.

care team providers. I hereby give consent to the case management services from (insert employer name or company name). I also understand I may terminate this consent at any time.

Patient signature: Witness and date:[17]

---

17. Ibid.

CHAPTER 7

CONCLUSION—READY, SET, GO

With any new nursing role, many find themselves wondering if they have made the right decision. Change is inevitable for most of us and happens in most careers. As with any change, avenues explode, which when properly nurtured, bring about a positive step in developing a person's career. Case management is definitely another avenue of nursing in which a nurse can expand the knowledge and skills mastered at the bedside into a whole new field of practice.

The bedside skills, clinical knowledge of disease processes, and routine treatment plans based on previous care plans or guidelines of practices will enhance your future oversight within the practice field of case management. Too often, nurses become frustrated within a few short months with second-guessing their career choices. They question if the choice they made is a good one.

Many nurses new to this field cannot really comprehend the nurse case manager role duties and the specifics related to the field until a year has passed. Give yourself ample time to prepare your mind for the long haul ahead.

For those who are good at mastering many activities, such as putting in long work weeks, managing family budgets, planning vacations, coordinating children's activities, and entertaining, this job change may be easy. Are you the person who has a passion for community involvement? If you fit into one of these categories, you may have one goal in mind.

That, my fellow nurse case manager, is to reach your greatest potential with the desired goals you've set for yourself. Reach your expectations and achieve a sense of assuredness in this challenging role.

Let me give you an important piece of advice to follow at this point in your new career choice. Simply take one day at a time, and recognize it may take five to ten years to perfect the skills necessary to be a nurse case manager.

Take a few moments to ask yourself the following questions and answer them honestly: Were you an expert as a bedside nurse within a few months of clinical practice? Did you have the answers to questions pertaining to practice specifics as a new graduate nurse? How long were you on orientation before you actually performed the duties expected?

Rome wasn't built in one day, and the skills necessary to perform case management duties will likely take a while to acquire as you become an effective nurse case manager.

Breathe in, breathe out, and take time to develop the community resource base and network with others proficient with job details. Ponder this: working at a snail's pace is better than running a rat race with no clear end in sight.

Immediately, you're thrown into a whole new world involving new terminology related to insurance and government programs. Expert communication skills are emphasized when dealing with the entire health team. This team consists of providers, insurance company representatives, nurses, caregivers, social services, patient advocates, therapists, nutritionists, and many other allied health team members.

Most of the language and verbiage centers upon patient care issues, enhancing patient safety, dismissal processes and plans, insurance requests, claims submitted, health plans, coding requests, contracts, government mandates, and facility policies, which in turn attempt to address and implement the utilization plan within the department. Check with the local library, institutional library center, or community organizations, or possibly seek out written policies related to this new avenue of career growth. Remember, snail's pace versus rat race.

It will take time, but eventually, you will become knowledgeable of basic case management practices. All of this involves dealing with insurance precertification and authorizations, working with providers, collaborating with health plans, mastering discharge planning processes, tapping into community resources, and so much more. Keep focused day by day on the task at hand.

The information presented in the previous chapters encompasses the role of the nurse case manager with tools for success, valuable tips, care planning processes, and basic utilization practice information. All this will surely guide you in your role in case management. Simply put, these are the basics of nursing case management.

You may find these tools valuable within various areas of this field of nursing. Case manager roles may differ according to the department model used. Hospital case management departments may indeed model their programs differently. The department model may hinge upon the size of the institution, average daily census, and budget restraints. Specific role delineation between a social worker and a case manager is clearly defined within the job description.

In some instances, the discharge planning may be left to the social workers while the case manager performs the utilization part. Concentrated efforts toward quality issues, tracking variances, and system problems are aligned with a dedicated nurse case manager's expertise. These efforts indeed help toward reaching the established institutional goals.

As you are aware, setting goals for yourself and for your family involves practice and a steady determination. Likewise, a supervisor establishes goals, and an employer will plan future goals. Sometimes, those in a position to make necessary changes need to think out of the box when formulating a desired plan toward achieving the desired outcomes set by the administrators of an institution.

Today, many corporations, including those in health care, are becoming more and more visionary toward future planning. Strategies to offset future government mandates are a top priority with administrators. Process changes are inevitable, and believe it or not, once you master a process change, it will change again.

Groups of individuals specialized in every aspect of a client's entry level for provider access meet in order to brainstorm ideas. Brainstorming allows all participants to engage in discussions. It is an opportunity to vocalize any problems or barriers perceived by both the client (as per feedback) and the institution.

Concerns regarding handling the dismissal planning part of patient care, preauthorization of scheduled procedures, patient medication assistance, and equipment needs top the list. A collaborative group of bedside nurses, physicians, nurse specialists, therapists, dieticians, and case managers combine their knowledge of process successes and failures in order to build upon future desired goals and improved outcomes. All efforts are centered on providing the best customer service for the patient.

Nurse case managers are a vital speaking component within these stages of planning. As Mullahy states, "Case managers are right in the center of activity as a force for change and as implementers of effective programs that have become our nation's response to the need for health care reform."[18] Their frontline knowledge of a patient's failed outpatient treatment plans and noncompliant issues help to identify key aspects in any concept of change.

Case management is a challenging but rewarding career. Bring the ideas, suggestions for improving processes, techniques,

18. C. M. Mullahy and D. K. Jensen, *Student Study Guide to Accompany The Case Manager's Handbook*, 3rd ed., p.101, (Sudbury, MA: Jones and Bartlett, 2004).

and skills that you've mastered at the bedside to connect with your patients in a new role, a role that encourages every nurse whether at the bedside or coordinating services to become the patient's advocate.

Helping a client with case management is truly exciting and benefits many parties involved. To those of you looking for a career change, please look into this alternative pathway of nursing. Congratulations to those entering this exciting field of nursing. Best wishes for an interesting and rewarding career as you embark upon the nurse case manager role.

About the Author

Charlotte Cox has worked in health care for over thirty years. She attained LPN status in 1977, graduated with an associate's degree in nursing from St. Mary's College of Nursing in O'Fallon, Missouri, in 1982, and finished her bachelor of science in nursing from Southwest Baptist University in 1996. Her nursing career included staff nursing in medical and intensive care units, as well as being an assistant nursing director of a cardiac step-down unit for many years.

She currently is the clinical case manager specializing in utilization and case management of cardiac patients and is the appeal coordinator for the utilization department. Charlotte is a certified case manager. Her current employment is with a large health system based in Southwest Missouri. Charlotte has penned numerous articles pertaining to nursing throughout her career.

Charlotte is a patient advocate and an active citizen frequently writing her elected officials with local and national health-care concerns. She readily admits that her nursing career is a blessing from the Lord.

Charlotte and her husband, David, reside in Southwest Missouri. They have three children (two daughters and a son) and enjoy family, friends, and the adventures of life.

DEFINITIONS AND TERMS RELATED TO UTILIZATION AND CASE MANAGEMENT

admission clinical review: Admission review of the medical record in which data is forwarded to the client's insurance company to explain the rationale for an acute inpatient hospital admission.

authorization or (certification): The approval of medical services, admission, or continued length of stay as determined by the insured's health plan with information provided.

avoidable days: Inpatient hospital days which possibly could have been avoided, attributable to a variety of issues, such as delays in testing or procedures, system issues related to timeliness of services rendered, physician consult delays, social issues, placement, or guardianship.

assisted living facility: (See also **independent living**) A facility that enables a person to live independently with available staff to help with meal preparation and personal care assistance and oversee medication dispensement for a designated daily, weekly, or monthly fee.

case management: A coordination of patient care delivery services that spans the entire health system access entry levels to ensure appropriate resources in meeting guidelines, timeliness concerns, and outcomes designated.

certified nurse case manager: A registered nurse who meets the requirements and has successfully obtained certification in the field of case management.

continued stay clinical review: A review in which the clinical data provided to the insurance supports the daily hospital stay.

contractual agreement: An agreement between parties based upon allowed charges in respect to claims submitted in accordance with health plan insurance polices.

denial: No authorization for health-care services in review of information provided.

disease management: A program designed to coordinate and manage specific groups of diseases with a focus on preventive measures, acute stages of care, and long-term maintenance of high-risk individuals.

heath maintenance organization (HMO): An organization that manages the health-care services needed for health plan members within a certain geographical area. A prefixed premium is paid as determined in providing quality services to the enrolled plan member.

home health care (HHC): An agency that provides health care in the home setting with skilled nursing, aide assistance, therapists, and social service assistance as outlined by the medical provider for a specified time. These services may be provided as private pay or as specified with the insurance according to the plan benefits.

homemaker care assistance: Assistance aimed at providing in-home services, such as grocery shopping, cleaning, cooking, errands, and sitter or companion needs, with a client remaining in the home environment. This service is provided by contracted agencies according to insurance benefit plans or private pay.

independent living or assisted living: Living arrangements to enhance the quality of life for persons who wish to remain as independent as possible with their health needs. Some facilities provide limited nursing services, meal preparation, laundry services, and medication assistance within a safe environment.

indigent: An individual with limited or nonexistent financial means to support the basic needs of life.

in-network: A predetermined health plan with contracted facilities, providers, and allied health professionals approved for delivery of care needs.

inpatient status: A hospital admission status determined on admission or during a continued hospital stay which usually meets with medical necessity guidelines.

length of stay: The number of days a patient is hospitalized within an acute care facility.

long-term assisted care facility (LTAC): An acute care facility that provides for an extended acute stay and rehabilitation to help meet the complex needs of an individual.

long-term care facility or nursing home: A facility designed to meet the needs of clients needing constant supervision of care needs that no longer can be provided in the home setting for an unspecified duration of time.

Medicaid: A federal public assistive program designed to give eligible individuals access to health care managed and operated by each state.

medical director: Designated physician who supervises and ensures that the quality of services rendered are in accordance with the utilization plan and the established guidelines and contractual agreements regarding the health plan.

Medicare: A federal insurance and supplementary program with coverage for hospital and outpatient services, prescriptions, medical equipment, and skilled facility and home health benefits to eligible elderly and disabled persons.

negotiation: To strike a deal between the health plan and providers of care in order to render services for a specified time with a specified set of terms.

National Provider Identification Number (NPI): A standardized identification of all providers who prescribe and refer cases in order to be paid by insurance companies.

nurse case manager: A registered nurse with designated specific skills and education requirements who practices within the field of case management.

nurse reviewer: A registered or licensed nurse who performs specific skills related to a departmental utilization plan as well as clinical reviews for insurance companies.

observation status: Designated hospitals short stay determination related to admission criteria guidelines.

out of network: Services provided to a health plan patient that are not in accordance with the approved in-network system providing delivery of care and services.

outpatient status: Designated hospitals short stay determination related to outpatient services of care provided.

physician advisor: The appointed advisor to the health-care team in the delivery of patient care and services in accordance with established facility guidelines.

point of service (POS): Health plans in which the client has a choice of providers but may pay increased deductibles, co-pays, or higher premiums in choosing a nonparticipating provider.

preferred provider organization (PPO): A program in which preferred providers are contracted to provide medical services to health plan participants.

precertification: Process to obtain approval of services from the health insurance company before services or procedures are performed.

retrospective clinical review: A documented clinical synopsis of care that is provided to the insurance company following services rendered or information collected for hospital management in review for providing quality services at reduced costs.

skilled nursing facility (SNF): A facility approved by Medicare that operates according to specific Medicare guidelines for admission of clients in helping to meet the skilled services required by nursing for a designated period of time.

social services: A department of educated, skilled employees equipped to guide and intervene with the social issues and identified needs of patients and families at the local or regional level.

third-party payer: A designated administrative group that handles claims and costs of care provided to the health plan members for an insurance group or health plan.

unavoidable days: Hospital patient days that usually are unavoidable, attributable to various identified issues within a health system or externally.

utilization plan: A departmental plan that outlines the departmental function and goals with specified outcomes in meeting with appropriate utilization and management of healthcare services within the health system. The utilization plan is supervised by a designated medical management team.

utilization management: Services reviewed to ensure medical necessity and quality and that such services are provided at the most appropriate level of entry in the health system.

variance days: Hospital patient days that usually are avoidable, attributable to various identified system issues. See **avoidable days**.

Complied list of terms taken from the following resources:

T. G. Cesta and H. A. Tahan, *The Case Manager's Survival Guide. Winning Strategies for Clinical Practice*, 2nd ed. (Philadelphia, PA: Mosby, 2003).

C. M. Mullahy and D. K. Jensen, *The Case Manager's Handbook*, 3rd ed. (Sudbury, MA: Jones and Bartlett, 2004).

REFERENCES

Case Management Society of America. "What Is a Case Manager?" http:/www.ccmcertification.org/ (accessed November 18, 2009).

————. 2006. *CMAG Case Management Adherence Guidelines.* Version 2.0. USA: Case Management Society of America.

Cesta, T. G., and H. A. Tahan. 2003. *The Case Manager's Survival Guide. Winning Strategies for Clinical Practice.* 2nd ed. Philadelphia, PA: Mosby.

Commission for Case Manager Certification. "Case Management Practice." http://www.ccmcertification.org/ (accessed November 18, 2009).

Daniels, S., and M. Ramey. 2005. *The Leader's Guide to Hospital Case Management.* Sudbury, MA: Jones and Bartlett Publishers.

Hale, D., and K. A. Bower. 2008. "Observation or Inpatient? Correct Patient Status More Critical than Ever." *Hospital Case Management* 16(6):81–84.

Huff, M. A, 2005. *Case Management Orientation, UR, UM and CM: The Basics.* Springfield, MO: St John's Mercy Hospital.

———. 2010. *Utilization Management Orientation.* Springfield, MO: St. Johns Mercy Hospital.

———. 2010. *Utilization Management. VA Denial Management.* Springfield, MO: St. John's Mercy Hospital.

Kongstvedt, P. R. 2004. *Managed Care, What It Is and How It Works.* 2nd ed. Sudbury, MA: Jones and Bartlett.

McKesson Corporation. 2009. *McKesson InterQual Level of Care Criteria.* Newton, MA: McKesson Corporation.

Milliman Care Guidelines. "Delivering Evidence-based Knowledge at the Point of Care." http://www.careguidelines.com/ (accessed April 19, 2010).

Mullahy, C. M., and D. K. Jensen. 2004. *The Case Manager's Handbook.* 3rd ed. Sudbury, MA: Jones and Bartlett.

———. 2004. *Student Study Guide to Accompany The Case Manager's Handbook.* 3rd ed. Sudbury, MA: Jones and Bartlett.

National Underwriter Company (The). 2006. *Tax Facts 2006 All About Medicare.* Cincinnati, OH: The National Underwriter Company.

Nightingale, F. 2003. *Notes on Nursing.* New York, NY: Barnes & Noble Books.

Poynter, D. 2007. *Dan Poynter's Self Publishing Manual. How to Write, Print and Sell Your Own Book.* 16th ed. Santa Barbara, CA: Para Publishing.

U.S. Department of Health & Human Services. "Centers for Medicare & Medicaid Services." http://www.hhs.gov (accessed December 22, 2007).

————. "Medicare, 5 Ways to Lower Your Costs during the Coverage Gap." http://www.hhs.gov (accessed December 22, 2007).